HBOT REJUVENATION

Total Healing for the Body with the magical powers of Hyperbaric Oxygen Therapy

Dr Sandra Moore

1. INTRODUCTION TO HYPERBARIC OXYGEN THERAPY

Hyperbaric oxygen therapy (HBOT) is a medical treatment that involves breathing pure oxygen in a pressurized environment. It has been used for decades to treat a variety of medical conditions and is based on the principle that increased atmospheric pressure can enhance the delivery of oxygen to tissues throughout the body.

History and Development

The roots of hyperbaric oxygen therapy can be traced back to the late 19th century when it was first explored as a treatment for decompression sickness, also known as "the bends," which affects divers who surface too quickly from deep dives. French physiologist Paul Bert conducted pioneering research in the late 1800s on the effects of increased atmospheric pressure and oxygen on living organisms.

In the early 20th century, hyperbaric chambers were developed to treat decompression sickness among divers and workers in high-pressure environments, such as caisson workers involved in underwater construction projects. These early chambers provided the foundation for the development of modern hyperbaric oxygen therapy.

During World War I and World War II, hyperbaric oxygen therapy gained further attention for its potential to treat wounds and infections in soldiers. Over the years, research and clinical experience have expanded the use of HBOT to include various medical conditions beyond decompression sickness and wound healing.

Basic Principles and Mechanisms of Action

Hyperbaric oxygen therapy works on the principle that increasing the pressure of the environment in which a person breathes oxygen can enhance the amount of oxygen dissolved in the bloodstream and delivered to tissues throughout the body. Under normal atmospheric pressure at sea level, the oxygen dissolved in the plasma of the blood is limited, but when exposed to increased pressure, more oxygen can be dissolved.

The increased oxygen delivery to tissues has several physiological effects, including:

- Improved oxygenation of hypoxic (oxygen-deprived) tissues, which can enhance wound healing and tissue repair.

- Reduction of tissue swelling and inflammation, which can alleviate pain and promote recovery from injuries.

- Stimulation of the body's natural defense mechanisms, including the immune system, to combat infections and support healing processes.

- Promotion of the formation of new blood vessels (angiogenesis) and the growth of new tissue (neovascularization), which can enhance tissue regeneration.

These mechanisms contribute to the therapeutic effects of hyperbaric oxygen therapy across a range of medical conditions, including wound healing, carbon monoxide poisoning, radiation injury, and certain neurological disorders.

In summary, hyperbaric oxygen therapy harnesses the power of increased atmospheric pressure and pure oxygen to enhance tissue oxygenation, promote healing, and support the body's natural healing processes. Understanding the history, principles, and mechanisms of action of HBOT is essential for appreciating its diverse applications in modern medicine.

2. UNDERSTANDING HYPERBARIC OXYGEN CHAMBERS

Hyperbaric oxygen chambers are specially designed enclosures that create a pressurized environment for administering hyperbaric oxygen therapy (HBOT). These chambers come in various types, each with its own features and capabilities, and understanding their design and function is crucial for safe and effective treatment delivery.

Types of Chambers

1. Monoplace Chambers: Monoplace chambers are designed to accommodate a single patient at a time. They are typically cylindrical or tube-like in shape and completely enclose the patient during treatment. Monoplace chambers are pressurized with pure oxygen, and the patient breathes this oxygen through a mask or hood. These chambers are suitable for most HBOT applications and are commonly found in hospitals and outpatient clinics.

2. Multiplace Chambers: Multiplace chambers are larger and can accommodate multiple patients simultaneously, along with healthcare

providers who administer treatment. These chambers are often used in hospital settings and are pressurized with compressed air, with patients breathing oxygen through masks or hoods. Multiplace chambers allow for more efficient use of space and resources, making them suitable for high-volume HBOT centers.

3. Portable Chambers: Portable hyperbaric chambers are smaller, inflatable units that can be set up in various locations, such as clinics, homes, or even on-site at remote locations. These chambers are pressurized with compressed air, and patients breathe

oxygen through a mask or hood. Portable chambers offer convenience and flexibility for patients who may have difficulty accessing traditional HBOT facilities.

4. Mild Hyperbaric Chambers: Mild hyperbaric chambers operate at lower pressures than traditional hyperbaric chambers, typically around 1.3 to 1.5 atmospheres absolute (ATA). They are often used for "mild" hyperbaric therapy, which is sometimes referred to as soft or low-pressure hyperbaric therapy. These chambers may use ambient air or oxygen-enriched air, and they are

primarily used for wellness and non-medical purposes.

How Hyperbaric Chambers Work

Hyperbaric chambers create a pressurized environment by either compressing ambient air or delivering pure oxygen at increased pressure. This increased pressure allows for the dissolution of a greater amount of oxygen in the bloodstream, which is then delivered to tissues throughout the body.

The operation of hyperbaric chambers involves several key components:

1. Pressure Vessel: The main chamber enclosure is typically made of metal or reinforced materials capable of withstanding high pressures. The design ensures airtightness and safety during pressurization.

2. Compression System: Monoplace chambers often use a compression system that delivers pure oxygen into the chamber to achieve the desired pressure. Multiplace chambers may use compressed air, which is pressurized by external compressors and delivered into the chamber.

3. Control Systems: Hyperbaric chambers are equipped with sophisticated control systems that regulate pressure, oxygen delivery, and other parameters during treatment. These systems ensure the safety and effectiveness of HBOT sessions and allow healthcare providers to monitor and adjust treatment parameters as needed.

4. Patient Interfaces: Patients receive oxygen during HBOT sessions through masks, hoods, or breathing tubes connected to the chamber. These interfaces ensure the delivery of oxygen-rich air to the patient's

respiratory system, promoting tissue oxygenation and therapeutic effects.

In summary, hyperbaric oxygen chambers come in various types and designs, each tailored to specific clinical needs and applications. Understanding how these chambers operate is essential for healthcare providers and patients to ensure safe and effective delivery of hyperbaric oxygen therapy.

3. CONDITIONS TREATED WITH HYPERBARIC OXYGEN THERAPY

Hyperbaric oxygen therapy (HBOT) has demonstrated efficacy in treating a wide range of medical conditions, leveraging the increased delivery of oxygen to tissues under pressure to promote healing and support various physiological processes. Let's delve into each of these conditions in detail:

1. Wound Healing:

Hyperbaric oxygen therapy is commonly used to facilitate wound healing in cases where traditional wound care approaches have been ineffective. By increasing oxygen delivery to the wound site, HBOT promotes angiogenesis (the formation of new blood vessels), enhances collagen production, and supports the body's natural immune response to infection. This makes it particularly effective in treating chronic, non-healing wounds such as diabetic foot ulcers, venous ulcers, and pressure sores.

2. Carbon Monoxide Poisoning:

Carbon monoxide (CO) poisoning occurs when individuals inhale toxic levels of carbon monoxide, often from sources such as faulty heating systems, vehicle exhaust, or fires. HBOT is utilized to rapidly eliminate carbon monoxide from the bloodstream and tissues by increasing the oxygen-carrying capacity of hemoglobin. This helps to restore tissue oxygenation and prevent long-term neurological damage associated with carbon monoxide poisoning.

3. Decompression Sickness:

Decompression sickness, also known as "the bends," occurs when divers ascend too quickly from deep dives, leading to the formation of nitrogen bubbles in the bloodstream and tissues. HBOT is the primary treatment for decompression sickness, as it increases ambient pressure, thereby reducing the size of nitrogen bubbles and promoting their elimination from the body. This helps alleviate symptoms such as joint pain, neurological deficits, and respiratory distress.

4. Radiation Injury

Radiation therapy is a common treatment for cancer, but it can also cause damage to surrounding healthy tissues and blood vessels, leading to complications such as radiation-induced fibrosis and necrosis. HBOT can mitigate these effects by promoting tissue oxygenation, reducing inflammation, and stimulating the growth of new blood vessels. This makes it an effective adjunctive therapy for managing radiation-induced injuries, particularly in cases of radiation cystitis, proctitis, and osteoradionecrosis.

5. Diabetic Ulcers:

Patients with diabetes are at increased risk of developing foot ulcers due to impaired wound healing and peripheral neuropathy. HBOT has been shown to improve wound healing in diabetic ulcers by enhancing tissue oxygenation, promoting angiogenesis, and increasing the activity of growth factors involved in the healing process. Additionally, HBOT can help reduce the risk of infection and amputation in patients with diabetic foot ulcers.

6. Traumatic Brain Injury:

Traumatic brain injury (TBI) can result in reduced blood flow and oxygenation to the brain, leading to neurological deficits and cognitive impairments. HBOT has shown promise as a treatment for TBI by increasing cerebral blood flow, reducing inflammation, and promoting neuroplasticity and neuronal repair.

While further research is needed to fully establish its efficacy, HBOT may offer benefits in improving cognitive function and quality of life in TBI patients.

7. Other Medical Conditions:

In addition to the conditions mentioned above, hyperbaric oxygen therapy has been investigated for its potential benefits in various other medical conditions, including:

- Crush injuries and compartment syndrome

- Gas gangrene

- Acute arterial insufficiency

- Non-healing surgical wounds

- Sudden sensorineural hearing loss

- Central retinal artery occlusion

- Multiple sclerosis

- Autism spectrum disorders

While the evidence supporting HBOT varies across these conditions, ongoing research continues to explore its therapeutic potential and refine treatment protocols for optimal patient outcomes.

In conclusion, hyperbaric oxygen therapy offers a versatile and effective approach to treating a wide range of medical conditions, leveraging the physiological benefits of increased tissue oxygenation under pressure. By understanding the mechanisms of action and clinical applications of HBOT, healthcare providers can optimize its use to improve patient outcomes and quality of life.

4. HYPERBARIC OXYGEN THERAPY PROCESS

Hyperbaric oxygen therapy (HBOT) is a systematic medical treatment that involves exposing patients to pure oxygen at increased atmospheric pressure inside a hyperbaric chamber. The therapy process typically consists of several key steps, including pre-treatment evaluation, adherence to treatment protocols, and determining the appropriate duration and frequency of treatments.

Pre-Treatment Evaluation:

Before undergoing hyperbaric oxygen therapy, patients undergo a comprehensive pre-treatment evaluation to assess their medical history, current health status, and suitability for HBOT. This evaluation involves:

1. Medical History: Healthcare providers review the patient's medical history, including any underlying medical conditions, previous surgeries, medications, allergies, and lifestyle factors that may affect treatment outcomes.

2. Physical Examination: A thorough physical examination is conducted to

assess the patient's overall health, vital signs, and any existing wounds or injuries that may benefit from HBOT.

3. Diagnostic Tests: Depending on the patient's condition and treatment goals, diagnostic tests such as blood tests, imaging studies (e.g., X-rays, MRI), and specialized assessments may be performed to gather additional information and guide treatment planning.

4. Informed Consent: Patients receive detailed information about the risks, benefits, and expected outcomes of HBOT, and they have the opportunity to

ask questions and provide informed consent before proceeding with treatment.

Treatment Protocols:

Once the pre-treatment evaluation is completed and the patient is deemed suitable for HBOT, healthcare providers develop individualized treatment protocols tailored to the patient's specific needs and medical condition. Treatment protocols may vary depending on factors such as the indication for HBOT, the severity of the condition, and the patient's response to therapy. Key aspects of treatment protocols include:

1. Pressure and Oxygen Levels: Treatment protocols specify the target pressure and oxygen concentration (e.g., 100% oxygen) to be used during HBOT sessions. These parameters are based on established clinical guidelines and may be adjusted based on the patient's response to therapy.

2. Session Duration: HBOT sessions typically last between 60 to 120 minutes, although shorter or longer sessions may be indicated based on the patient's tolerance and treatment goals. The number of sessions prescribed varies

depending on the condition being treated and the desired therapeutic outcomes.

3. Compression and Decompression Phases: Patients undergo gradual compression to reach the desired treatment pressure inside the hyperbaric chamber, followed by a period of oxygen breathing at pressure (compression phase). After the treatment session is completed, the chamber is gradually depressurized (decompression phase) to allow patients to safely return to normal atmospheric pressure.

Duration and Frequency of Treatments:

The duration and frequency of hyperbaric oxygen therapy treatments vary depending on the patient's condition, treatment goals, and response to therapy. In general:

1. Acute Conditions: Patients with acute conditions such as carbon monoxide poisoning or decompression sickness may require a short course of HBOT consisting of one or a few sessions to rapidly eliminate toxins or gas bubbles from the body and alleviate symptoms.

2. Chronic Conditions: Patients with chronic conditions such as chronic

wounds, radiation injuries, or diabetic ulcers may require multiple HBOT sessions over several weeks to months to achieve optimal healing and long-term therapeutic benefits. Treatment frequency may range from once daily to several times per week, with periodic reassessment of progress and treatment adjustments as needed.

3. Maintenance Therapy: In some cases, patients may benefit from maintenance or intermittent HBOT to sustain therapeutic effects and prevent disease recurrence. Maintenance therapy schedules are typically less frequent than initial treatment regimens and are

individualized based on the patient's response to therapy and ongoing medical needs.

In summary, the hyperbaric oxygen therapy process involves a comprehensive pre-treatment evaluation, adherence to individualized treatment protocols, and careful consideration of the duration and frequency of treatments to optimize therapeutic outcomes and ensure patient safety and well-being. Collaboration between healthcare providers and patients is essential throughout the treatment process to monitor progress, address any concerns, and achieve the best possible results.

5. BENEFITS AND RISKS OF HYPERBARIC OXYGEN THERAPY

Hyperbaric oxygen therapy (HBOT) offers a range of potential benefits for patients across various medical conditions, but like any medical intervention, it also carries certain risks and side effects. Understanding the balance between benefits and risks is crucial for healthcare providers and patients when considering the appropriateness of HBOT for individual cases.

Potential Benefits:

1. Enhanced Wound Healing: HBOT promotes tissue oxygenation and angiogenesis, leading to accelerated wound healing in conditions such as diabetic ulcers, venous ulcers, and non-healing surgical wounds.

2. Improved Oxygen Delivery: By increasing the oxygen-carrying capacity of blood and tissues, HBOT can enhance oxygenation in hypoxic (oxygen-deprived) tissues, supporting healing processes and reducing inflammation.

3. Treatment of Decompression Sickness: HBOT is highly effective in treating

decompression sickness ("the bends") by reducing the size of nitrogen bubbles in the bloodstream and promoting their elimination from the body.

4. Management of Carbon Monoxide Poisoning: HBOT rapidly eliminates carbon monoxide from the bloodstream, preventing tissue hypoxia and neurological damage associated with carbon monoxide poisoning.

5. Radiation Injury Management: HBOT mitigates the effects of radiation-induced tissue damage by promoting tissue oxygenation, reducing inflammation, and supporting wound healing in conditions

such as radiation cystitis, proctitis, and osteoradionecrosis.

6. Neurological Benefits: HBOT has shown promise in improving outcomes in traumatic brain injury (TBI) by increasing cerebral blood flow, reducing inflammation, and promoting neuroplasticity and neuronal repair.

Possible Side Effects and Risks:

1. Barotrauma: Rapid changes in pressure during compression and decompression phases of HBOT can cause barotrauma, leading to ear pain,

sinus discomfort, or, in rare cases, barotrauma to the lungs or other organs.

2. Oxygen Toxicity: Prolonged exposure to high levels of oxygen can lead to oxygen toxicity, causing symptoms such as seizures, vision changes, or respiratory distress. This risk is minimized by carefully controlling treatment parameters and duration.

3. Fire Hazard: Oxygen-rich environments inside hyperbaric chambers increase the risk of fire, particularly in the presence of flammable materials or electrical equipment. Strict

safety protocols are in place to minimize this risk.

4. Claustrophobia: Some patients may experience feelings of claustrophobia or anxiety while inside the hyperbaric chamber, particularly in monoplace chambers that fully enclose the patient.

5. Middle Ear Barotrauma: Changes in pressure during HBOT can cause middle ear barotrauma, leading to ear pain, hearing loss, or eardrum rupture. Techniques such as equalizing pressure and ear protection devices can help mitigate this risk.

6. Sinus Barotrauma: Pressure changes can also cause sinus barotrauma, resulting in sinus pain, congestion, or sinusitis. Patients with pre-existing sinus conditions may be at increased risk.

CONTRAINDICATIONS:

1. Untreated Pneumothorax:
Patients with untreated pneumothorax (collapsed lung) should not undergo HBOT due to the risk of worsening the condition.

2. Uncontrolled Seizure Disorders: Patients with uncontrolled seizure disorders may be at increased risk of

oxygen toxicity during HBOT and should be carefully evaluated before treatment.

3. Certain Medications: Some medications, such as certain chemotherapeutic agents or certain drugs that interfere with oxygen delivery (e.g., doxorubicin), may interact with HBOT and increase the risk of side effects or complications.

4. Certain Respiratory Conditions: Patients with certain respiratory conditions, such as chronic obstructive pulmonary disease (COPD) or severe asthma, may be at increased risk of

complications during HBOT and should be evaluated on a case-by-case basis.

In summary, hyperbaric oxygen therapy offers potential benefits for a wide range of medical conditions but also carries certain risks and side effects that must be carefully considered and managed. Healthcare providers play a critical role in assessing patient suitability for HBOT, monitoring treatment parameters, and mitigating potential risks to ensure safe and effective therapy outcomes.

RESEARCH AND EVIDENCE SUPPORTING HYPERBARIC OXYGEN THERAPY

Hyperbaric oxygen therapy (HBOT) has been the subject of extensive research and clinical trials over several decades, providing valuable insights into its mechanisms of action, efficacy, and safety profile across various medical conditions. Here, we explore the wealth of evidence supporting HBOT's therapeutic benefits and its effectiveness in treating diverse health conditions.

Clinical Studies and Trials:

1. Wound Healing: Numerous clinical studies have demonstrated the efficacy of HBOT in promoting wound healing, particularly in chronic and non-healing wounds such as diabetic ulcers, venous ulcers, and pressure sores. Randomized controlled trials (RCTs) have shown significant improvements in wound closure rates, reduction of wound size, and prevention of amputations in patients undergoing HBOT compared to standard wound care alone.

2. Carbon Monoxide Poisoning: HBOT is considered the standard of care for the treatment of carbon monoxide poisoning, supported by robust clinical evidence

from RCTs and observational studies. These studies have consistently shown faster elimination of carbon monoxide from the bloodstream, reduced incidence of neurological sequelae, and improved outcomes in patients receiving HBOT compared to normobaric oxygen therapy.

3. Decompression Sickness: The effectiveness of HBOT in treating decompression sickness has been well-established through both clinical trials and real-world experience in hyperbaric medicine centers worldwide. RCTs have demonstrated faster resolution of symptoms, improved neurological outcomes, and reduced

morbidity and mortality rates in divers and individuals experiencing decompression sickness following hyperbaric oxygen treatment.

4. Radiation Injury: HBOT has shown promise in managing radiation-induced tissue injuries, including radiation cystitis, proctitis, and osteoradionecrosis. Clinical studies and case series have reported significant improvements in symptom relief, wound healing, and quality of life in patients receiving HBOT as adjunctive therapy to conventional treatments such as surgery or radiation therapy.

5. Traumatic Brain Injury: While the evidence for HBOT in traumatic brain injury (TBI) is still evolving, several clinical trials and observational studies have suggested potential benefits in improving neurological function, cognitive outcomes, and quality of life in TBI patients. Ongoing research aims to further elucidate the mechanisms of action and optimal treatment protocols for HBOT in TBI management.

Effectiveness in Various Conditions:

Beyond the conditions mentioned above, HBOT has demonstrated efficacy and therapeutic potential in a wide range of medical conditions, including:

- Diabetic Ulcers: HBOT has been shown to improve wound healing and reduce the risk of amputation in patients with diabetic foot ulcers, particularly in cases of non-healing or infected wounds.

- Gas Gangrene: HBOT is effective in treating gas gangrene, a potentially life-threatening bacterial infection of soft tissues, by promoting tissue oxygenation and inhibiting bacterial growth.

- Sudden Sensorineural Hearing Loss: HBOT has been investigated as a treatment for sudden sensorineural hearing loss, with some studies suggesting improved hearing outcomes when HBOT is initiated early in the course of the condition.

- Multiple Sclerosis: HBOT has shown promise in managing symptoms and improving quality of life in patients with multiple sclerosis, although further research is needed to establish its long-term efficacy and optimal treatment protocols.

In summary, hyperbaric oxygen therapy has garnered substantial research support and clinical evidence for its effectiveness across a spectrum of medical conditions, ranging from wound healing and carbon monoxide poisoning to radiation injury and traumatic brain injury. Continued research efforts aim to expand our understanding of HBOT's therapeutic mechanisms and refine treatment protocols to maximize patient outcomes and improve healthcare delivery.

7. INTEGRATING HYPERBARIC OXYGEN THERAPY INTO HEALTHCARE

Integrating hyperbaric oxygen therapy (HBOT) into healthcare involves collaboration among healthcare providers, ensuring accessibility to patients, and addressing financial considerations such as insurance coverage and reimbursement. Here's an in-depth exploration of these aspects:

Collaborating with Healthcare Providers:

1. Multidisciplinary Approach: Effective integration of HBOT into healthcare requires collaboration among various healthcare providers, including hyperbaric medicine specialists, wound care specialists, primary care physicians, surgeons, and allied health professionals. A multidisciplinary approach ensures comprehensive patient care and optimal treatment outcomes.

2. Referral and Consultation: Primary care physicians and specialists may refer patients to hyperbaric medicine centers for evaluation and treatment. Collaboration between referring providers and hyperbaric specialists

involves exchanging relevant medical information, discussing treatment goals, and coordinating care throughout the HBOT process.

3. Interdisciplinary Case Conferences: Interdisciplinary case conferences provide a platform for healthcare providers to discuss complex cases, share expertise, and formulate individualized treatment plans for patients receiving HBOT. These conferences promote communication, collaboration, and shared decision-making among members of the healthcare team.

4. Continuing Education and Training: Healthcare providers involved in the delivery of HBOT undergo specialized training and continuing education to ensure proficiency in treatment protocols, safety procedures, and patient management. Ongoing training programs and professional development opportunities support the delivery of high-quality care and promote best practices in hyperbaric medicine.

Insurance Coverage and Reimbursement:

1. Insurance Coverage: Many health insurance plans provide coverage for

hyperbaric oxygen therapy when medically necessary and prescribed by a qualified healthcare provider. Coverage may vary depending on the patient's insurance plan, the specific medical condition being treated, and the guidelines established by insurance carriers.

2. Prior Authorization: Prior authorization from the insurance company may be required before initiating HBOT to confirm medical necessity and ensure coverage eligibility. Healthcare providers submit documentation, including clinical indications, diagnostic tests, and

treatment plans, to support the request for prior authorization.

3.   Reimbursement   Policies: Reimbursement for hyperbaric oxygen therapy is governed by reimbursement policies established by insurance carriers, Medicare, and other third-party payers. These policies outline coverage criteria, billing codes, documentation requirements, and reimbursement rates for HBOT services.

4. Coding and Documentation: Healthcare providers use specific Current Procedural Terminology (CPT) codes to bill for hyperbaric oxygen therapy

services, along with appropriate diagnosis codes to indicate the medical necessity of treatment. Accurate and comprehensive documentation of patient encounters, treatment sessions, and outcomes is essential for successful reimbursement and compliance with insurance guidelines.

5. Appeals Process: In cases where insurance claims for HBOT services are denied or partially denied, healthcare providers may appeal the decision through the insurance company's appeals process. Appeals typically involve submitting additional documentation, clinical rationale, and supporting

evidence to justify the medical necessity of HBOT and request reconsideration of the claim.

In summary, integrating hyperbaric oxygen therapy into healthcare involves collaboration among healthcare providers, adherence to insurance coverage and reimbursement policies, and a commitment to delivering high-quality, evidence-based care to patients. By fostering interdisciplinary collaboration and navigating the complexities of insurance reimbursement, healthcare providers can ensure that patients have access to the benefits of HBOT as part of their comprehensive treatment plans.

8. PATIENT EXPERIENCES AND TESTIMONIALS

Patient experiences and testimonials play a crucial role in understanding the impact of hyperbaric oxygen therapy (HBOT) on individuals' lives. By sharing their personal stories, patients provide valuable insights into the effectiveness, benefits, and challenges associated with HBOT. Here, we explore some common themes and experiences shared by individuals who have undergone HBOT:

Healing and Recovery:

1. Wound Healing: Many patients who have undergone HBOT for chronic wounds, diabetic ulcers, or radiation injuries report significant improvements in wound healing and tissue regeneration. They often describe how HBOT helped them avoid amputation, reduce pain, and regain mobility, improving their overall quality of life.

2. Symptom Relief: Patients with conditions such as carbon monoxide poisoning, decompression sickness, or sudden sensorineural hearing loss often share stories of symptom relief and rapid recovery following HBOT. They describe how HBOT helped alleviate symptoms

such as headache, dizziness, fatigue, and hearing loss, allowing them to return to normal activities sooner.

3.   Neurological Improvement: Individuals with traumatic brain injury (TBI) or neurological disorders may experience cognitive improvements, mood stabilization, and enhanced functional abilities after undergoing HBOT. They may report clearer thinking, improved memory, and better concentration, contributing to greater independence and well-being.

Quality of Life:

1. Pain Management: Patients with chronic pain conditions, such as fibromyalgia, complex regional pain syndrome (CRPS), or musculoskeletal injuries, may find relief from pain and discomfort through HBOT. They often share how HBOT sessions helped reduce pain levels, improve sleep quality, and enhance overall comfort and well-being.

2. Improved Energy and Vitality: Some patients undergoing HBOT for general wellness or non-specific health concerns report feeling more energized, rejuvenated, and mentally alert after treatment sessions. They may describe increased vitality, enhanced physical

stamina, and a greater sense of vitality and resilience.

3. Emotional Well-being: HBOT can have positive effects on emotional well-being, mood regulation, and stress management. Patients may share how HBOT helped them feel calmer, more relaxed, and better able to cope with stress, anxiety, or depression, leading to greater emotional balance and resilience.

Challenges and Considerations:

1. Time Commitment: Patients undergoing HBOT often discuss the time commitment involved in completing

multiple treatment sessions over several weeks or months. They may need to allocate time for transportation to and from the hyperbaric facility and adjust their schedules to accommodate treatment appointments.

2. Financial Considerations: Some patients may face financial barriers to accessing HBOT, particularly if insurance coverage is limited or unavailable for their specific medical condition. They may need to explore alternative funding options or seek assistance from healthcare providers or charitable organizations.

3. Adjustment to the Chamber: Patients may initially feel apprehensive or claustrophobic when entering the hyperbaric chamber, particularly in monoplace chambers that fully enclose the patient. However, with guidance and support from healthcare providers, many patients adapt to the chamber environment and become more comfortable with subsequent treatments.

In summary, patient experiences and testimonials provide valuable insights into the real-world impact of hyperbaric oxygen therapy on individuals' lives. By sharing their stories of healing, recovery, and quality of life improvement, patients contribute to greater awareness, understanding, and appreciation of the benefits of HBOT within the healthcare community and beyond.

9. FUTURE DIRECTIONS AND INNOVATIONS IN HYPERBARIC OXYGEN THERAPY

Hyperbaric oxygen therapy (HBOT) continues to evolve as researchers explore new applications, refine treatment protocols, and develop innovative technologies to enhance its efficacy, safety, and accessibility. Here, we delve into the exciting future directions and emerging trends in HBOT:

Emerging Research Areas:

1. Neurological Disorders: Ongoing research aims to elucidate the potential

benefits of HBOT in treating neurological conditions such as stroke, traumatic brain injury (TBI), Alzheimer's disease, and Parkinson's disease. Preliminary studies suggest that HBOT may promote neuroplasticity, reduce inflammation, and improve functional outcomes in patients with various neurological disorders.

2. Chronic Inflammatory Conditions: HBOT is being investigated as a potential treatment for chronic inflammatory conditions such as rheumatoid arthritis, Crohn's disease, and inflammatory bowel disease. By modulating immune responses, reducing inflammation, and

promoting tissue repair, HBOT may offer therapeutic benefits in managing these challenging conditions.

3. Cancer Therapy Support: HBOT is being explored as an adjunctive therapy to conventional cancer treatments, including radiation therapy and chemotherapy. Research suggests that HBOT may enhance tumor oxygenation, sensitize cancer cells to radiation and chemotherapy, and reduce treatment-related side effects such as radiation-induced tissue damage.

4. Regenerative Medicine: HBOT holds promise in regenerative medicine

applications, including tissue engineering, wound healing, and organ transplantation. By stimulating angiogenesis, enhancing stem cell mobilization, and promoting tissue regeneration, HBOT may accelerate healing and improve outcomes in regenerative medicine interventions.

Technological Advancements:

1. Advanced Hyperbaric Chambers: Technological advancements in hyperbaric chamber design and construction aim to improve patient comfort, safety, and treatment efficacy. Innovations such as integrated

monitoring systems, adjustable seating, and enhanced ventilation systems enhance the patient experience and optimize treatment delivery.

2. Hyperbaric Oxygen Delivery Systems: Novel hyperbaric oxygen delivery systems, including mask designs, breathing apparatus, and oxygen delivery methods, are being developed to improve oxygen delivery efficiency, minimize waste, and enhance patient convenience. These innovations ensure optimal oxygenation during HBOT sessions and support patient compliance with treatment protocols.

3. Hyperbaric Monitoring and Imaging: Advanced monitoring technologies and imaging modalities are being integrated into hyperbaric chambers to provide real-time feedback on patient physiology, oxygenation levels, and tissue responses during HBOT. Non-invasive monitoring techniques such as near-infrared spectroscopy (NIRS) and tissue oxygenation monitors offer insights into tissue perfusion and oxygen delivery, guiding treatment optimization and individualized care.

4. Hyperbaric Telemedicine: Telemedicine platforms and remote monitoring systems enable healthcare

providers to remotely assess and monitor patients undergoing HBOT, enhancing access to care and facilitating collaboration among multidisciplinary teams. Telemedicine consultations, virtual follow-up visits, and remote monitoring of treatment parameters optimize patient management and support continuity of care.

In summary, the future of hyperbaric oxygen therapy is marked by exciting research advancements and technological innovations that promise to expand its therapeutic potential, improve treatment outcomes, and address unmet medical needs across a broad spectrum of health conditions. By embracing emerging research areas and leveraging cutting-edge technologies, HBOT continues to evolve as a valuable tool in modern medicine, offering hope and healing to patients worldwide.

10. CONCLUSION

Hyperbaric oxygen therapy (HBOT) has emerged as a versatile and effective medical intervention with applications across a wide range of health conditions. As we conclude our exploration of HBOT, let's summarize the key points and reflect on the future of this innovative therapy:

Summary of Key Points:

1. Mechanism of Action: HBOT involves exposing patients to pure oxygen at increased atmospheric pressure, leading to enhanced oxygen delivery to tissues, improved wound healing, reduced

inflammation, and other therapeutic effects.

2. Clinical Applications: HBOT is utilized in the treatment of diverse medical conditions, including chronic wounds, carbon monoxide poisoning, decompression sickness, radiation injuries, diabetic ulcers, traumatic brain injury, and more.

3. Efficacy and Safety: Extensive research and clinical evidence support the efficacy and safety of HBOT in promoting healing, relieving symptoms, and improving outcomes for patients across various health conditions.

4. Integration into Healthcare: Integrating HBOT into healthcare involves collaboration among healthcare providers, adherence to insurance coverage and reimbursement policies, and a commitment to delivering high-quality, evidence-based care to patients.

5. Patient Experiences: Patient experiences and testimonials provide valuable insights into the real-world impact of HBOT, highlighting the benefits of healing, symptom relief, and improved quality of life observed by

individuals who have undergone treatment.

6. Future Directions: Emerging research areas and technological advancements in HBOT hold promise for expanding its therapeutic potential, addressing unmet medical needs, and enhancing treatment outcomes across a broad spectrum of health conditions.

Final Thoughts on the Future of Hyperbaric Oxygen Therapy:

The future of hyperbaric oxygen therapy is bright, with ongoing research efforts and technological innovations driving advancements in treatment efficacy, safety, and accessibility. As we look ahead, several key trends and developments shape the trajectory of HBOT:

1. Personalized Medicine: Advances in precision medicine and individualized treatment approaches enable healthcare providers to tailor HBOT protocols to each patient's unique needs, optimizing therapeutic outcomes and minimizing risks.

2. Interdisciplinary Collaboration: Collaborative efforts among healthcare providers, researchers, and industry

stakeholders foster innovation and drive progress in HBOT, leading to the development of new treatment modalities, delivery systems, and clinical applications.

3. Expanding Clinical Indications: Continued research into the mechanisms of action and therapeutic effects of HBOT expands its clinical indications, opening new avenues for treatment in areas such as neurology, oncology, regenerative medicine, and chronic disease management.

4. Technological Advancements: Advances in hyperbaric chamber design,

oxygen delivery systems, monitoring technologies, and telemedicine platforms enhance the efficiency, safety, and accessibility of HBOT, improving patient experiences and outcomes.

5. Global Access: Efforts to increase global access to HBOT through education, training, infrastructure development, and policy advocacy ensure that patients worldwide can benefit from this life-saving therapy, regardless of geographic location or socioeconomic status.

In conclusion, hyperbaric oxygen therapy represents a cornerstone of modern medicine, offering hope and healing to patients facing a wide range of health challenges. By embracing emerging research areas, leveraging technological innovations, and fostering interdisciplinary collaboration, the future of HBOT holds immense potential to transform healthcare delivery, improve patient outcomes, and advance human health and well-being. As we continue to unlock the mysteries of oxygen under pressure, the journey of discovery in hyperbaric medicine promises to yield new insights, innovations, and breakthroughs that shape the future of healthcare for generations to come.

GLOSSARY OF TERMS:

1. Hyperbaric Oxygen Therapy (HBOT): A medical treatment that involves breathing pure oxygen in a pressurized environment, typically inside a hyperbaric chamber, to promote healing and provide therapeutic benefits.

2. Monoplace Chamber: A hyperbaric chamber designed to accommodate one patient at a time, fully enclosing the patient within the chamber during treatment.

3. Multiplace Chamber: A hyperbaric chamber designed to accommodate

multiple patients simultaneously, typically with a larger chamber volume and windows for observation and communication.

4. Decompression Sickness: A condition resulting from rapid changes in pressure, often experienced by divers ascending too quickly, leading to the formation of nitrogen bubbles in the bloodstream and tissues.

5. Carbon Monoxide Poisoning: Toxic exposure to carbon monoxide gas, typically from sources such as faulty heating systems, vehicle exhaust, or fires,

leading to tissue hypoxia and neurological symptoms.

6. Wound Healing: The physiological process of repairing damaged tissues and restoring skin integrity following injury, surgery, or disease.

7. Radiation Injury: Tissue damage caused by exposure to ionizing radiation, commonly associated with cancer treatments such as radiation therapy.

8. Traumatic Brain Injury (TBI): A form of brain injury resulting from external mechanical force, leading to cognitive

impairments, neurological deficits, and functional disabilities.

9. Angiogenesis: The process of new blood vessel formation from pre-existing vessels, essential for wound healing, tissue repair, and oxygen delivery to tissues.

10. Neuroplasticity: The brain's ability to reorganize and adapt in response to injury, learning, or environmental changes, facilitating recovery and functional adaptation.

Frequently Asked Questions (FAQs):

1. What conditions can be treated with hyperbaric oxygen therapy?

Hyperbaric oxygen therapy is used to treat a variety of medical conditions, including wound healing, carbon monoxide poisoning, decompression sickness, radiation injuries, diabetic ulcers, traumatic brain injury, and more.

2. How does hyperbaric oxygen therapy work?

HBOT involves breathing pure oxygen in a pressurized environment, typically inside a hyperbaric chamber. This increases the oxygen concentration in the bloodstream, promoting tissue oxygenation, reducing inflammation, and supporting healing processes.

3. Is hyperbaric oxygen therapy safe?

HBOT is generally considered safe when administered by trained healthcare professionals in appropriate clinical settings. However, there are potential risks and side effects associated with HBOT, including barotrauma, oxygen toxicity, and ear or sinus discomfort.

4. How many hyperbaric oxygen therapy sessions are needed?

The number and frequency of HBOT sessions vary depending on the patient's condition, treatment goals, and response to therapy. Patients may undergo a series of treatments over several weeks or months, with periodic reassessment of progress and treatment adjustments as needed.

5. Is hyperbaric oxygen therapy covered by insurance?

Many health insurance plans provide coverage for HBOT when medically necessary and prescribed by a qualified healthcare provider. Coverage criteria, prior authorization requirements, and reimbursement policies vary depending on the patient's insurance plan and specific medical condition.

These resources and FAQs serve as valuable references for patients, caregivers, and healthcare professionals seeking information, support, and guidance on hyperbaric oxygen therapy and related topics.